CW00831964

Coconut Oil:

Coconut Oil for Beginners - 33 Amazing Coconut Oil Recipes for Hair Care, Natural Beauty, Anti-Aging and Beautiful Soft Skin!

TABLE OF CONTENTS

Introduction

Coconut oil has been used for thousands of years on a daily basis, not only in food preparation but also for beauty. As from recent years, it has created a sudden boom in the beauty world for its many benefits for reducing cellulite, moisturizing dry hair and skin, and many other properties.

So what is this miracle oil? Coconut oil is an edible oil extracted from the kernel or meat of mature coconuts harvested from the coconut palm. It contains saturated fats which help promote one's heart health and weight loss (where needed) and also support your immune system along with other benefits.

However, this book deals with only its cosmetic properties and recipes. When applied to the skin the saturated fats in the coconut oil absorb and continue to hold the moisture content of the skin, as the fats eliminate moisture loss.

Lauric acids have strong disinfectant and anti-microbial properties, so when applied to the skin, coconut oil protects it from infections which can enter the body through open wounds, and any other external bacteria threats.

Like coconuts themselves, coconut oil is very protein rich. These proteins keep skin healthy and revitalized, on the inside, and out. Proteins also contribute to cellular health and tissue repair, along with a wide range of other essential activities within the body. All of this also goes for hair, since coconut oil treatment significantly reduces protein loss from either damaged or undamaged hair.

Now let's take a look at all the different ways you can incorporate this oil into healthy alternatives for your usual beauty products.

Chapter 1: Coconut Oil for Hair

Lavender and Coconut Oil Hairspray

This natural alternative will not have the same strong hold of the alcohol-laden hairsprays. Instead the coconut oil will help reduce frizzing while also hydrate and strengthen your hair. Lavender oil gives a soothing, relaxing and refreshing feel to your tresses, which makes this spray perfect for hot, summer days.

Ingredients:

- 2 tbsp. of coconut oil
- 3-4 drops of lavender essential oil
- 2 c. water (distilled)
- a spray bottle

Instructions:

Melt the coconut oil using a double boiler (if you do not have one, simply add water into a saucepan, put it on high temperature and place a glass bowl over the water) or microwave and add to spray bottle along with the distilled water and essential oil and shake the bottle. The ingredients will not combine permanently, separation is normal so make sure you shake the bottle well before each use. Spritz on damp or dry hair. You can add different essential oils depending on what you prefer (peppermint or rosemary are great alternatives).

Deep Hair Conditioner

Deep conditioning helps remove any toxins caused by the chemicals in hair products and repair the damage caused by sun or sea water. The combination of coconut oil, argan oil and shea butter makes this conditioner perfect for dry and frizzy hair. It moisturizes your hair, adds shine and helps control frizzing while also protecting it from UV rays. Either of the essential oils (lavender, peppermint or rosemary) help soothe and relax your hair.

Ingredients:

- 2 tbsp. of coconut oil
- 1 tbsp. of shea butter
- 1 tsp. of Argan oil
- A couple of drops of essential oil (either peppermint, lavender or rosemary work great for hair)

Instructions:

Melt coconut oil and shea butter together in microwave or double broiler (if you do not have one, simply add water into a saucepan, put it on high temperature and place a glass bowl over the water). Let the mixture cool slightly then add Argan oil and essential oil (you can use all three if you like) and whip together for 3-5 minutes. Comb through clean, dry hair and let sit for 30 minutes. Rinse the conditioner out of your hair with lukewarm water and shampoo it as usual.

Protein Treatment for Curly Hair

This DIY protein-pack is guaranteed to help bring the bounc-
iness back to your lifeless curls. Coconut oil provides your
hair follicles with both hydration and protection from UV
rays. The egg yolk offers your hair the proteins that keep
your hair strong and help it grow.

Ingredients:

- a tbsp. of coconut oil
- 2 eggs

Instructions:

Take the 2 eggs and separate the egg yolks from the whites.
Mix the egg yolk with 1 tbsp. of coconut oil. Soak your hair
with the mixture and leave it on for about 40 minutes.

Use the egg whites to cleanse your scalp from any dry skin
cells. Before rinsing make sure you have set the water to cool
or you will cook the protein-pack in your hair.

Honey and Coconut Oil Hair Treatment

The combination of coconut oil and honey help moisturize and bring shine to your hair leaving it soft and silky to the touch. The egg yolks provide the hair with the necessary proteins for strengthening your hair.

Ingredients:

- 3 tbsp. of coconut oil
- 1.5 tbsp. of honey
- 2 egg yolks (optional)
- a heated towel
- essential oil for fragrance (optional)

Instructions:

Melt the coconut oil in microwave or double boiler (if you do not have one, simply add water into a saucepan, put it on high temperature and place a glass bowl over the water) for a couple of minutes. Pour the melted coconut oil into a bowl, add the honey and mix. This is when you add the essential oil of your preference if you wish. Apply the mixture to wet hair from ends to roots and wrap a warm towel over your hair (if you add the egg yolks skip this step so that they do not cook in your head). After 45 minutes, rinse out your hair.

Hair Growth Oil

Ingredients:

- 2-3 tbsp. of coconut oil
- a tbsp. of argan oil
- 1-2 tbsp. of olive oil

Instructions:

Mix all of the ingredients and melt them in a microwave or double boiler (if you do not have one, simply add water into a saucepan, put it on high temperature and place a glass bowl over the water). Apply the mixture and massage it onto your scalp for 5 minutes. Leave it for 4 hours, (best to do it overnight) and put a shower cap or plastic bag over your hair. After 4 hours, or after you wake up, shampoo your hair as usual.

Hair Tonic

This hair tonic is great if you need to refresh your dry hair or manage your misbehaving strands. It can also be used before styling as a hair sheen.

Ingredients:

- 1/3 c. of melted coconut oil
- 1 c. of water (filtered)
- a tsp. of vodka
- 8 drops of jasmine essential oil
- a spray bottle

Instructions:

Mix the melted coconut oil with the filtered water into the spray bottle. Then add a teaspoon of vodka and jasmine essential oil and shake well. You can also replace jasmine with lavender or rosemary oil, or any other of your choice. Make sure you shake the spray bottle well before each use.

Chapter 2: Coconut Oil for Skin

Whipped Body Butter

The combination of coconut oil, shea butter and jojoba oil in this body butter provides your skin with protection against harmful UV rays, infections and bacteria, while at the same time moisturizing it. Lavender essential oil leaves your skin with a soothing and relaxing feel.

Ingredients:

- ½ c. of coconut oil
- 1 c. of shea butter
- ½ c. of jojoba oil
- 10 drops of lavender essential oil

Instructions:

Melt the oils together using a double boiler (if you do not have one, simply add water into a saucepan, put it on high temperature and place a glass bowl over the water) which will make them semi-clear when ready or a microwave. Then put the mixture in the refrigerator until it becomes solid. Using a mixer, whip the oils until they are the same texture as whipped cream. Add the essential oil (peppermint essential oil is a great alternative) and mix to combine. Pour it into a container of your choice and refrigerate for an hour. Apply the butter after taking a shower for the best results.

Coconut Oil Lavender Salt Scrub

This recipe combines the energizing effects of sea salt with the moisturizing effects of coconut oil that leave the skin feeling smooth and refreshed. The drops of lavender oil offer a soothing and relaxing feeling to your skin as well as remove any toxins and dead skin cells from your skin.

Ingredients:

- 2 c. of coconut oil
- 1 c. of sea salt
- 20 drops of lavender essential oil (chamomile does the trick, too)

Instructions:

Put the coconut oil, sea salt and lavender essential oil into a bowl and stir them until well combined. Pour the mixture into a container with an airtight lid and store in the fridge until ready to use. Scrub the mixture into your skin in circular motions until the salt dissolves. Rinse your skin out with lukewarm water and dap to dry.

Hand Scrub

While the salt and sugar help exfoliate the skin, the coconut oil and honey moisturize it. Together they leave the skin soft and smooth to the touch. The lemon juice helps lighten the skin and remove any odors (especially ones caused by garlic or onions).

Ingredients:

- 2 tbsp. of coconut oil
- 4 tbsp. of raw honey
- ½ c. of sea salt
- ½ c. of unrefined sugar
- 2 tbsp. of lemon juice

Instructions:

Mix the honey with the coconut oil in a bowl. In a different bowl, blend the salt, sugar and lemon juice. Pour the salt mixture into the honey mixture and stir until it becomes smooth. Place it into a small glass jar. Apply the scrub on your hands like you were washing them with soap. Do this until the salt and sugar have dissolved then wash it off with lukewarm water. Do this 2-3 times a week.

Coconut Oil Lotion Bar

The combination of coconut oil and beeswax make this lotion bar a perfect replacement for a moisturizer. It helps reduce dryness of the skin and bring back its softness and springiness (characteristics of well-nourished and hydrated skin). The addition of eucalyptus and peppermint essential oils gives your skin protection from inflammations and a soothing feeling.

Ingredients:

- 1 c. of coconut oil
- 3/4 c. of pure beeswax
- a few drops of eucalyptus and peppermint essential oils (optional)

Instructions:

Melt the coconut oil and beeswax together in a microwave or double boiler (if you do not have one, simply add water into a saucepan, put it on high temperature and place a glass bowl over the water). After the coconut oil and beeswax have melted add the essential oils and combine well. Pour the mixture into silicone bar molds or muffin molds. Leave the lotion to cool for a few hours; if you like you can speed up the process by putting it in the refrigerator for an hour. Before using, warm the bar up until it is soft enough to apply to your skin and rub it on clean skin. Depending on what your skin needs you can change the essential oils.

Shaving Cream

The combination of coconut oil, shea butter and almond oil make this recipe perfect for sensitive skin, prone to skin irritations and ingrown hairs. It will not only help the razor glide smoothly over your skin but also leave it feeling soft and moisturized. Additionally, chamomile essential oil helps provide the skin with a soothing feeling.

Ingredients:

- 4 tbsp. of shea butter
- 3 tbsp. of coconut oil
- 2 tbsp. of almond oil
- 10-12 drops of chamomile essential oil (optional)

Instructions:

Melt the shea butter and coconut oil using a microwave or double boiler (if you do not have one, simply add water into a saucepan, put it on high temperature and place a glass bowl over the water). Once combined, remove from heat. Add the almond oil and chamomile essential oil (lavender works well, too) and mix them in to combine. Then let the mixture cool in the refrigerator. After it hardens, using a mixer whip the mixture until it looks like whipped cream. Let it rest for 5 minutes and then pour it into an airtight container. Store them in the fridge when you are not using them.

Deodorant for Sensitive Skin

This deodorant is simple and is an excellent alternative for people who no longer want to use the toxin-filled products on the market. Coconut oil provides the skin with all the nutrients it needs as well as hydration, leaving the skin smooth. Rosemary and peppermint essential oils help sooth your skin while also refreshing it. Keep in mind that this is not an antiperspirant.

Ingredients:

- 1/3 c. of coconut oil
- 2 tbsp. of baking soda
- 1/3 c. of arrow root powder
- 10 drops of rosemary essential oil
- 5 drops of peppermint essential oil

Instructions:

Mix the coconut oil, baking soda and arrow root powder in a small mixing bowl. Combine the ingredients until it resembles the consistency of a deodorant. Add in the essential oils stir well to combine. Place the mixture in a small container of your choice. Apply it two minutes before dressing to avoid smearing on your clothes.

Sunscreen Lotion Bars

The combination of coconut oil, beeswax, shea butter and vitamin E oil provides your skin with the same amount of SPF protection without any of the unhealthy ingredients contained in the store-bought lotions. The addition of rosemary essential oil gives your skin a relaxing feel and also repels any bug bites, especially mosquitoes.

Ingredients:

- ½ c. coconut oil
- 5 tbsp. beeswax
- ½ c. of shea butter
- 2 tbsp. zinc oxide
- ½ tsp. vitamin E oil
- ¾ tsp. rosemary essential oil
- a silicone mold

Instructions:

Melt the shea butter, coconut oil and beeswax using a double boiler (if you do not have one, simply add water into a saucepan, put it on high temperature and place a glass bowl over the water) until completely combined. Remove from the heat and mix in our zinc oxide, essential oil and the vitamin E oil. Place the mixture into a silicone mold and refrigerate for half an hour to cool. After they have hardened remove the bars from the mold. When going sunbathing keep the bar away from the sunshine or they will melt and make a mess.

Chapter 3: Coconut Uses for Your Face

Cleansing Face Oil for Sensitive Skin

The combination of coconut oil, milk powder and honey help provide the skin with hydration and works wonders on sensitive skin. The addition of rose water helps sooth and cool sensitive and irritated skin. Honey will also protect your skin from harmful UV rays.

Ingredients:

- 4 tbsp. of coconut oil
- 3 tbsp. of milk powder
- 1 c. of rose water
- 1 tbsp. of honey

Instructions:

In a bowl mix the milk powder with rose water. Using a microwave or a double boiler, or if you do not have one, simply add water into a saucepan, put it on high temperature and place a glass bowl over the water, melt the coconut oil. Once it is melted, add it to the mixture along with the honey. Pour the mixture into a bottle and store it in the fridge. Make sure you shake it well before you use it.

Cleansing Cream for Dry Skin

The combination of coconut oil and egg yolk help provide the skin with necessary proteins that keep it hydrated. Apple cider vinegar is great for dealing with acne-prone skin removing the layer of dead skin cells and leaving the complexion brighter.

Ingredients:

- 1 egg yolk
- 1 tbsp. of apple cider vinegar
- ½ tsp. of sugar
- 8 tbsp. of coconut oil
- A few drops of essential oils (optional)

Instructions:

Mix the egg yolk with apple cider vinegar and sugar and combine well. Gradually add in the coconut oil while constantly stirring, like when making mayonnaise. Once it has a creamy texture, pour it into a jar, or any other container of your choice. Store it in your fridge. Apply a thin coat of the cream in circular motions onto your face. Leave it to soak into your skin for 10 minutes and rinse it out with lukewarm water.

Lemon Honey and Coconut Oil Face Mask

The combination of coconut oil and honey helps hydrate the skin and reduce acne scarring. The acids in lemon juice help tighten the skin and brighten the skin tone as well as kill any bacteria from your skin.

Ingredients:

- a tbsp. of coconut oil
- ½ tbsp. of lemon juice
- 2 tsp. of honey
- A drop of lavender essential oil (optional)

Instructions:

Mix the coconut oil, lemon juice and honey (and essential oil if you want) together in a small bowl. Make sure combine them well. Then apply a thick layer of the mixture onto you face and let the skin soak it in for about 10 minutes. When the time has passed rinse the mask off with cold water. Replace the lavender oil with chamomile, they have similar properties.

Coconut and Almond Oil Cleanser

This cleanser is perfect for fighting off the dry cold winter air. The combination of coconut and almond oil helps moisturize the skin and acts anti-inflammatory. Cocoa butter offers the skin with properties that fight off free radicals (molecules, usually caused by exposure to pollution and UV rays, which can affect cellular processes).

Ingredients:

- 3 tbsp. of coconut oil
- 1 ½ tbsp. of olive oil
- 2 tsp. of cocoa butter
- 5 tsp. of sweet almond oil
- 20 drops of jasmine essential oil

Instructions:

Melt the coconut oil with the cocoa butter in a microwave or a double boiler (if you do not have one, simply add water into a saucepan, put it on high temperature and place a glass bowl over the water). Mix them together and let them cool. After the mixture cools, add the almond oil and olive oil and keep on mixing. Let it cool a while, add in the jasmine essential oil and combine it well. Pour the mixture in jars or any other container of your choice and store them in the fridge.

Acne Spot Treatment

The combo of coconut and tea tree oil is perfect since both have anti-bacterial and anti-fungal properties which help fight off bacteria and reduce redness.

Ingredients:

- ¼ c. of coconut oil
- 10 drops of tea tree essential oil
- lip balm tubes

Instructions:

Melt the coconut oil in a microwave or a double boiler (if you do not have one, simply add water into a saucepan, put it on high temperature and place a glass bowl over the water) and then add the tea tree essential oil. Combine it completely. You can use an eye dropper to pour it into the lip balm tubes. Place them in the refrigerator so as they do not melt. Make sure your face is clean before applying it.

Coconut Oil Facial Scrub

This face scrub can be used not only to clean your face but also to clean your entire body. It can replace your make-up remover and moisturizer due to the many benefits of coconut oil. While the sugar helps remove any dead skin cells and leaves the skin feeling smooth, the essential oils help refresh and relax your skin.

Ingredients:

- 3 c. of unrefined sugar
- 1 c. of brown sugar
- 1 c. of coconut oil
- A few drops of jasmine and peppermint essential oils

Instructions:

Melt the coconut oil in a microwave or a double boiler (if you do not have one, simply add water into a saucepan, put it on high temperature and place a glass bowl over the water). Mix sugar into the melted coconut oil. Then add the essential oils to the bowl and combine well. Pour the mixture into any container of your preference and store it in the fridge.

Turmeric Coconut Oil Face Mask

The combination of coconut oil and turmeric helps fight off acne and pimples, thanks to their anti-inflammatory properties. Turmeric also balances out uneven complexion and the banana removes acne scars and hydrates the skin.

Ingredients:

- 1 tbsp. of coconut oil
- ½ of a ripe banana
- ½ tsp. of turmeric

Instructions:

Mash up the ripe banana and add the coconut oil and turmeric. Stir until it is completely combined. Apply the mixture onto your face (make sure it is clean) and leave it on for 15 minutes. Remove it with cool water.

Avocado Coconut Oil Face Mask

This mask will leave your skin soft and hydrated also without having to spend too much. Coconut oil and avocado moisturize and nourish your skin as nutmeg helps to exfoliate the skin and protect against acne.

Ingredients:

- 1 tbsp. of coconut oil
- ¼ of a ripe avocado
- ½ tsp. of nutmeg

Instructions:

Peel the avocado, put it in a bowl and mash it into a smooth paste. Add the coconut oil and nutmeg and mix until combined completely. Apply a thick layer of the mixture onto your face and leave it on for about 15 minutes. Rinse it off with cool water.

Honey Coconut Oil Face Mask

While the coconut oil moisturizes the skin and the honey heals and softens it, the tea tree essential oil preserves and detoxifies the skin. The lavender essential oil protects the skin from any inflammations and acne.

Ingredients:

- 2 tbsp. of coconut oil
- 1 tbsp. of raw honey
- a drop each of lavender and tea tree essential oils

Instructions:

Stir the coconut oil with the raw honey. After it is well-mixed add the essential oils and mix it until it is completely combined. Apply a thin layer of this mixture onto your skin in circular motions, and let it soak into the skin for 10 minutes. Rinse it off with cool water or remove it with a warm towel.

Chapter 4: Coconut Oil Uses for Lips

Lip Sugar Scrub

The coconut oil helps moisturize your lips and provides protection against the elements. White and brown sugar help exfoliate the skin and remove any dead skin cells. Mint extract leaves a soothing and refreshing feeling on your lips, while also removing bacteria.

Ingredients:

- 3 tsp. of coconut oil
- 2 tbsp. of white sugar
- 4 tbsp. of brown sugar
- ½ tsp. of mint extract

Instructions:

Mix the two sugars in a small bowl and stir in the coconut oil. Add mint extract and after it is well combined put it in small containers (little glass jars are best). If you would like you can first melt the coconut, but make sure you add it slowly into the sugar. You can also replace the mint extract with either vanilla or lavender, or any other of your choice.

Chocolate Lip Scrub

The combo of coconut and vitamin E oil leave the skin moisturized and hydrated. Brown sugar acts as a great exfoliator, and helps remove the dead skin cells from your lips. Cocoa powder is rich is anti-oxidants which fight off free radicals (molecules, usually caused by exposure to pollution and UV rays, which can affect cellular processes).

Ingredients:

- 3 tbsp. of coconut oil
- 6 tbsp. of brown sugar
- 3 drops of vitamin E oil
- 1 tbsp. of unsweetened cocoa powder

Instructions:

First combine the brown sugar and unsweetened cocoa powder and then stir in the coconut oil and vitamin E oil. After mixing it thoroughly, pour it into a small container of your choice. Make sure you store them in the fridge to make them last longer. If you like you could also add a teaspoon of coffee powder.

Coconut Vanilla Lip Balm

Jojoba, beeswax and coconut oil provide the skin with hydration simultaneously protecting your lips from the sun, wind, dry air and other elements. Vanilla extract gives this lip balm a nice surprise element not to mention the amazing smell.

Ingredients:

- 3 tbsp. of coconut oil
- 1 c. of beeswax
- 1 tsp of vanilla extract
- 1 tsp of jojoba oil

Instructions:

Shave off a cup of beeswax and melt it with the coconut oil using a double boiler (if you do not have one, simply add water into a saucepan, put it on high temperature and place a glass bowl over the water). After they have melted mix in the jojoba oil and vanilla extract. Once all of the ingredients are combined pour the mixture into your containers. You can always replace the vanilla with any other extract; coconut, peppermint and lavender are among some great choices.

Coconut Rose Lip Balm

Apart from providing the skin with hydration and sun protection, like beeswax, coconut and olive oil, shea butter is an excellent source of vitamin A, E and F. Rose essential oil helps the skin fight off any inflammations and has a relaxing and refreshing effect.

Ingredients:

- 1/8 c. of coconut oil
- ¼ c. of beeswax
- 1/8 c. of shea butter
- 1 tsp. of vanilla extract
- 1 tsp. of virgin olive oil
- A few drops of rose essential oil

Instructions:

Using a double boiler (if you do not have one, simply add water into a saucepan, put it on high temperature and place a glass bowl over the water) melt the coconut oil and shea butter, stir in the olive oil and vanilla extract. After it is combined well, add the rose essential oil. Store the mixture in small containers of your choice. If you like you can add a few rose petals for esthetic effect.

Tinted Coconut Lip Balm

With the combination of beeswax, coconut and sweet almond oil, this lip balm is perfect for chapped and dry lips caused by either dry, cold winter air or dry, hot summer air. It offers both hydration and sun protection. Lavender oil provides a soothing and calming effect on lips.

Ingredients:

- 2 tbsp. of beeswax (shaved)
- 1 tbsp. of coconut oil
- 2 tsp. of almond oil
- a piece of red lipstick
- a couple of drops of lavender essential oil

Instructions:

Melt the beeswax, coconut oil, almond oil and lipstick using a double boiler (if you do not have one, simply add water into a saucepan, put it on high temperature and place a glass bowl over the water). Make sure you don't overcook them. After they are combined thoroughly, remove the mixture from heat and add lavender essential oil. Then pour it into small containers of your choice. If you would like it to be harder and balmy, so as to use it like a chap stick, then increase the amount of beeswax.

Chocolate Mint Lip Balm

Coconut oil, cocoa butter, vitamin E oil and almond oil help moisturize the lips and protect them from harmful UV rays. The combination of almond and vitamin E oil is perfect for helping the skin fight off free radicals (molecules, usually caused by exposure to pollution and UV rays, which can affect cellular processes).

Ingredients:

- 1 tbsp. of coconut oil
- 1 tbsp. of sweet almond oil
- 1 tbsp. of cocoa butter
- 9-10 drops of vitamin E oil
- 3-4 drops of peppermint essential oil
- 9-10 semisweet chocolate chips

Instructions:

Melt all the ingredients in a double boiler (if you do not have one, simply add water into a saucepan, put it on high temperature and place a glass bowl over the water) and mix them well. After a few minutes, pour the mixture into a sterilized small container. Make sure you store them in dark and cool place. Try not to put them in direct contact with sunlight or heat, or else they will melt.

Peppermint Lip Balm

While the coconut oil, beeswax and cocoa butter help moisturize chapped and dry lips with their emollient properties, they also prevent UV rays from harming the skin cells. Vitamin E oil prevents skin damage from free radicals (molecules, usually caused by exposure to pollution and UV rays, which can affect cellular processes) and the peppermint provides a cooling sensation.

Ingredients:

- 1/2 c. of coconut oil
- ½ c. of beeswax
- ½ c. of cocoa butter
- a few drops of vitamin E oil
- a few drops of peppermint essential oil
- lip balm tubes

Instructions:

Melt the coconut oil, beeswax and cocoa butter using a double boiler (if you do not have one, simply add water into a saucepan, put it on high temperature and place a glass bowl over the water). After the ingredients are completely combined, add the vitamin E and peppermint essential oil. Then pour the mixture into the lip balm tubes and let them cool for an hour or so. If you want a softer balm double the amount of coconut oil.

Chapter 5: Coconut Oil – Other Uses

Coconut Oil Pulling

Coconut oil pulling is a great way for removing bacteria and promoting healthy teeth and gum. It helps detoxify the oral cavity. This method has been used to clean teeth for thousands of years, and through recent research it has proven to stop tooth decay and loss, kill bad breath and many others. The addition of peppermint oil in this recipe gives a refreshing aftertaste.

Ingredients:

- 1-2 tbsp. of coconut oil
- A drop of peppermint essential oil

Instructions:

Mix the coconut oil together with the peppermint oil. Put it in your mouth and swish it around for 10-20 minutes (start with 10 minutes for your first time then slowly work yourself up). After you are done, spit the oil out into the trashcan (never into the sink since coconut oil will solidify and clog your sink). Then rinse out your mouth with salt water and brush your teeth as usual. Make sure you do this immediately after waking up.

Oil Pulling

Coconut oil pulling is a great way for removing bacteria and promoting healthy teeth and gum. It helps detoxify the oral cavity. This method has been used to clean teeth for thousands of years, and through recent research it has proven to stop tooth decay and loss, kill bad breath and many others. The addition of oregano oil in this recipe further helps refresh your breath and clean your teeth.

Ingredients:

- 1-2 tbsp. of coconut oil
- 1-2 drops of oregano essential oil

Instructions:

Mix the coconut and oregano oil together. Put the mixture into your mouth and swish for about 10-20 minutes (when starting out do it for 10 minutes the slowly work up) while also making sure you do not swallow any of the mixture. Then spit the oil out of your mouth (spit it into a trash can, not sink) and rinse it out with salt water a few times. Afterwards, brush your teeth as usual. Make sure you do this immediately after waking up. Repeat this 4 times a week for ultimate results.

Healing Coconut Oil Salve

The combination of yarrow flowers, calendula flowers, comfrey leaves, plantain leaves and rosemary leaves with coconut oil is perfect for fighting against any skin irritations, inflammations and also for speeding up the healing of wounds, cuts, bruises or burns. This salve is also naturally antibiotic, anti-fungal and astringent.

Ingredients:

- 1 ½ c. of coconut oil
- ¼ c. beeswax (shaved)
- 2 tbsp. of dried comfrey leaves
- 2 tbsp. of dried plantain leaves
- 1 tbsp. of dried calendula flowers
- 1 tsp. of dried yarrow flowers
- 1 tsp. of dried rosemary leaves

Instructions:

Infuse the herbs with the coconut oil. There are two ways to do this. One way to do this is to heat the herbs and coconut oil low heat in a double boiler for about 3 hours, which is far quicker than the second. The other way of infusing is mixing the herbs with almond oil in a jar and leaving it in the sun for 3-4 weeks, checking it daily. You can use almond oil instead. After you have infused the herbs, strain them out of the oil using a cheesecloth or strainer and throw away the herbs. Warm the oil up with beeswax until it is combined and pour the mixture into lip balm tubes, jars or any other container of your choice.

Herb Infused Coconut Oil

The combination of yarrow flowers, calendula flowers, comfrey leaves and marigold flowers with coconut oil is perfect for fighting against any skin irritations, inflammations and also for speeding up the healing of wounds, cuts, bruises or burns. Tea tree, lavender and rosemary essential oils fight off bacteria while also soothing the skin. This salve is also naturally antibiotic, anti-fungal and astringent.

Ingredients:

- 2-3 c. of coconut oil
- 4 tbsp. of dried yarrow flowers
- 4 tbsp. of dried calendula flowers
- 4 tbsp. of dried comfrey leaves
- 4 tbsp. of dried marigold flowers
- 1 oz. of beeswax per 8 oz. of herbal infused oil
- A few drops of tea tree, lavender and rosemary essential oil

Instructions:

Infuse the herbs with the coconut oil. The quickest way to do this is to heat the herbs and coconut oil low heat in a double boiler for about 3 hours. After you have infused the herbs, strain them out of the oil using several layers of cheesecloth, butter muslin or a tea towel that you do not mind staining. Make sure you get all the oil out and throw away the herbs. Warm the oil up with beeswax until it is combined and remove it from heat before you add the essential oils. Once the mixture is completely combined, pour it into lip balm tubes, jars or any other container of your choice.

Conclusion

So that brings us to the end of this recipe book. As it has already been mentioned coconut oil provides the hydration and rejuvenates the skin. It is an almost miracle-working oil and there is little this oil cannot do.

Whether it be your skin, hair or even your teeth, coconut oil has all it takes to fix any problems you might have. From dry skin to bruises it is a remedy for everything.

However, please note that like with all things, coconut oil should be used in moderation. There is a chance that if you do not apply it in thin layers on your skin when using it as a moisturizer it could clog your pores. So make sure you do not overdo it.

And finally, have fun with making these products and remember that you can always put your own twist on them. Being creative with these recipes might help you later create your own recipes.

Printed in Great Britain
by Amazon.co.uk, Ltd.,
Marston Gate.